LIFESTYLE

2000

Secrets of Natural Living
For the 21st Century

Mark & Ernestine Finley

ISBN 1-882846-00-1

Contents

Nutrition and Your Health

Situated on top of a cliff overlooking the emerald blue waters of the Mediterranean is an ancient Portuguese monastery. The view is breathtaking. The scenery is magnificent. But there is one problem. The only way to get to the top of the cliff is in an old wicker basket tied to a rope and hoisted up by an aged monk.

One day a guide and visitor were leaving the monastery. As they stepped into the basket and were lowered down by the monk, the rope swung out over the jagged rocks below. Nervously the tourist asked, "How often do they replace the rope?" "Don't worry," the guide replied in a reassuring tone, "every time one breaks, we replace it."

Just as in this story, thousands of people place themselves in an unpredictable situation regarding their health. They wait until their health snaps, like the rope, then frantically grasp onto the latest health fad. Broken health is not as easily replaced as a snapped rope! Health is not a matter of chance, it is a matter of choice — of obedience to nature's laws.

In the following pages we shall present scientifically proven, common-sense, and widely accepted principles of nutrition. You will discover how to prepare healthy, delicious, and well-balanced meals that will bring enjoyment to the table and may add years to your life now and into the 21st century.

The wise old saying, "It is better to prevent disease than to cure it," truly makes common sense, doesn't it? Isn't it much better to prevent disease by eating right and living right, and following proper health principles, than to allow the rope to snap? Isn't it much better to safeguard our health than to recklessly run through life, violating the very laws of our being, predisposing ourselves to heart disease, cancer, and an early death?

A hundred years ago infectious diseases were the major killers in the western world. By infectious diseases, we mean diseases such as pneumonia, tuberculosis, influenza; those diseases that are largely spread by germs, bacteria, or viruses.

While some infectious diseases are making a comeback in the latter part of the 20th century, a radical change is occurring. The leading killers are now degenerative diseases, such as heart disease, cancer, and arteriosclerosis. These are diseases of our lifestyle, diseases that we are bringing upon ourselves.

Although this may not seem like good news, degenerative diseases associated with lifestyle choices mean that there are factors within our control that will enable us to reduce the risk of these diseases. *Six out of ten leading causes of death in America are diet-related.* The United States Government became so concerned about nutrition and health that the Senate established a Select Subcommittee on nutrition. The committee carefully researched nutritional issues facing the Western World today. It attempted to analyze the diet of Americans, and to evaluate the relationship between poor diet and disease. The leading experts in the area of health throughout the U.S. pooled their knowledge. The leading research centers in America combined to bring the latest scientific research to the Senate Subcommittee. Hundreds of research projects were brought together. The conclusion: According to the Senate Select Committee on Human Needs, improved nutrition could cut the nation's health bill by one third!

During this century, the American diet has gone through an amazing transformation. Natural carbohydrates (fruits, vegetables, grains, and beans), which were once the mainstay of the American diet, now play a secondary role. Fat and sugar consumption have risen to the point where they comprise at least 40% of the American diet. This is an amazing reversal. In the early 1900s, fruits, nuts, grains, and vegetables (carbohydrates) were part of the mainstay of the American diet. But today, all this has changed.

In this book we're not going to launch into some kind of faddish approach to diet. Our goal is not to put you on carrot sticks for the rest of your life. Neither will we be telling you that if you progress to the absolute state of perfection in diet, you'll eat nothing more than rice. You may enjoy carrot sticks, and you may even enjoy rice. We do. But we're not going to put you on a diet that in any way is bizarre, extreme, or unscientific. We're rather going to focus on some basics, essentials. Here are our six major goals:

1. Increasing the natural foods in the diet.
2. Reducing overall fat consumption.
3. Reducing sugar consumption.
4. Replacing flesh meats with vegetarian proteins.

5. Increasing the overall amount of fiber and whole grains in the diet.
6. Learning how to make tasty, well-prepared natural food dishes.

As you implement these dietary principles, you will live longer, feel better and experience greater happiness.

The first area of emphasis is whole grains, dietary fiber and "Homemade Breadmaking Made Easy." Somebody has said: "Bread is the staff of life." Yet a Redbook magazine survey of 85,000 women indicated that only one in ten women bake their own bread regularly. The same survey revealed the fact that 45% never use any unrefined or natural foods such as whole wheat flour, brown rice, soy beans, honey, or granola.

Advantages of Making Homemade Bread

From a health perspective, are there good reasons to make your own homemade bread? Why take the time and energy when you can easily go to the store and simply buy it? What are the advantages of good homemade bread? Is white bread as nutritiously healthy as whole grain bread? What about the enriching process — doesn't that solve the problem? When some of the vitamins and minerals are taken out of the whole grain, aren't they added back? These are some good questions. Let's explore some answers.

Whole grain breads are an excellent source of dietary fiber. Fiber is the portion of vegetable cellular material left after digestion. It provides cellulose or roughage in the diet. Breads like French breads, Italian breads, and traditional white breads, do not have dietary fiber in any quantity.

Fiber is an extremely important part of the diet, because it assists in preventing the big three killers: heart disease, cancer, and stroke. In those countries where there is a high-fiber diet, there is also reduced heart disease and cancer. In countries where there is a low-fiber diet, we find a high incidence of heart disease, cancer, and stroke.

Researchers, for example, have studied the Japanese culture. They discovered that Japanese living in rural areas have a diet that is very high in fiber. Whole grain rice and vegetables comprise a large portion of their diet. This high-fiber diet, combined with a low-cholesterol diet, places them in an excellent preventive position for coronary heart disease. So those Japanese living in rural areas have very little coronary heart disease.

When the Japanese move to the cities and adopt a diet that is lower in fiber and much higher in fat, their heart disease rate goes up. When they move to Hawaii, and adopt the diet that is more westernized, their heart disease rate goes up even higher. But when those same Japanese families move to the United States, and live in San Francisco, for example, eating a diet that is extremely high in fat, very highly refined, and very low in fiber, their heart disease goes still higher.

Whole grain breads are an excellent source of B-vitamins. B-vitamins assist in stabilizing the nervous system. Where diets are low in the B-complex vitamins, particularly Thiamine, individuals tend to be more nervous, more anxious, more irritable and tense. When the diet is higher in Vitamin B, the individual tends to be more even-tempered. Significant scientific studies have confirmed this repeatedly. Whole grain breads have the natural goodness as packaged

5

by our loving Creator. They are not depleted by processing and then artificially enriched.

Someone has asked, "Doesn't the enrichment process add back everything that was taken away?" Maybe I can illustrate it this way. Let's suppose that you laid down your purse, and I carefully opened it, took out your wallet, and robbed you of $20. Later on, I began to feel quite guilty because I had robbed you. As the result of that, I came up to you and said, "Look, I'm sorry about taking $20 from you. I'd really like to give you $4 back." Would you feel enriched? You wouldn't, would you! Why not? I've just given you $4! But you would say, "Wait a minute, you stole $20 from me, and you're giving me $4 back. I'm not enriched; I've lost $16!"

Well, the enrichment process adds back at least four essential nutrients to depleted white flour: thiamine, riboflavin, niacin, and iron. Those are three important vitamins and an important mineral. But 16 others generally are not "paid back." Some of these additional 16 may play a significant role in health maintenance.

Dr. Rodger J. Williams, from the University of Texas, called attention to the deficiencies of enriched white flour over 20 years ago in a speech before the National Academy of Science in the fall of 1970. He described experiments with rats who were fed only commercially-enriched white flour. Within 70 days, 45 of the original 66 rats were dead of malnutrition.

You might say, "Who's going to only eat commercially-enriched white flour? We eat other things besides that." That's not the point. What we're trying to determine is the comparison of white flour and whole wheat flour. Obviously, you're going to eat more than white flour, or more than whole wheat flour. We're not saying that white flour is going to kill you — at least not immediately. We are saying that it predisposes you to diseases, and whole wheat flour helps in the prevention of those diseases.

In a group of 64 rats fed bread made of white flour supplemented with additional vitamins and minerals (plus lysine, an amino acid essential to growth), all but three gained weight and thrived. Those rats fed on the whole grain bread did well. Whole grains in their natural packaging are an important ingredient to health.

Whole grain breads are free from some of the artificial preservatives and additives which may be present in commercially-prepared breads. More and more researchers are concerned about artificial preservatives and additives. We should make a distinction between additives and preservatives. A preservative is something that is added to the bread, often natural, not chemical, to preserve either flavor, or to keep the bread from decaying. It retards spoiling. Additives are generally added for color or taste. Most of the time they are chemicals. Any time you add chemical substances to food, you run the risk of predisposing the body to disease.

Here's more good news! Homemade whole grain breads are much cheaper! In an age when the economy is soft and we're having difficulty making our house and car payments, we need all of the extra resources possible. The average loaf of homemade whole grain bread costs 65 cents. The average loaf of whole grain store-bought bread costs $1.55, more than twice as much. That is quite a bit more per loaf, and the monthly difference in bread alone for a family of five is $27. That would indicate about a $320 difference every year.

Somebody said, "Don't look a gift horse in the mouth." You'd have to work a number of hours to make $320. Although finance is not the main reason, it certainly is a good reason to adopt a lifestyle in which we make our own homemade bread.

Another great reason to make good homemade bread is that whole grain breadmaking is a lost art in today's fast-paced society; it provides a sense of family cohesiveness and security. More than once, driving up the road to my house on a hot summer day, feeling tense and anxious, I have smelled that beautiful aroma of homemade bread wafting up from our home. And I've said to myself, "I'm so happy I have a wife who makes homemade bread. Not only do I love that aroma, but I love to eat it, too!"

So here are six good reasons to make homemade bread. Let's review them:

1. Whole grain breads are an excellent source of dietary fiber.
2. They are also a great source of Vitamin B.
3. They're not depleted by processing.
4. They do not have artificial preservatives and additives.
5. Homemade bread is inexpensive.
6. Homemade bread brings the family together.

Isn't that worth it? Doesn't that inspire you to make your own whole grain bread?

Diet and Disposition

Diet affects not only our physical health, but our mental health as well. Studies indicate that a good diet with adequate whole grains significantly influences behavior. Several people who testified at a recent hearing of the United States Select Committee on Nutrition and Human Needs offered the opinion that what one eats is likely to affect one's behavior and mental health. Diet even assists in rehabilitating criminals. Barbara Reed, Chief Probation Officer in Cuyahoga Falls, Ohio, affirmed that when criminals are switched from junk foods (which are usually high in sugar) to fruits, foods high in protein, complex carbohydrates such as vegetables and whole grains, and vitamin supplements, their return rate to court after being released from jail is much lower than those who continue to eat mostly junk foods.

Carolyn Brown, Executive Director of a residential facility for delinquent children in Berkeley, California, testified that in her opinion there is a direct connection between juvenile delinquency, disturbed children, and nutrition. She didn't say that good nutrition is the total answer to the problems involved in juvenile delinquency and disturbed children. But she did argue that a diet free of chemicals, low in refined carbohydrates, free of synthetic foods, with a judicious and individualized program of nutritional supplementation, together with the avoidance of foods and chemicals that destroy health, promotes a positive mental attitude. Carolyn Brown summarized her statement before the Senate Subcommittee with these words: "There is a direct connection between a wholesome, nutritious diet and a lowered crime rate."

George Watson wrote a book called *Nutrition and Your Mind.* One of the illustrations in the book pictures two women. The first lady has a grouchy look on her face; her hair is all messed up and disheveled. She is sloppily dressed.

Watson pictures her sitting at a table. On a plate before her there are french fries, a hamburger, and a milk shake, apple pie, and ice cream — a diet that is obviously high in fat and high in sugar.

Then he pictures a lady who looks quite different. She is sitting at the table with a great big smile on her face; her hair is well kept, her clothing very becoming, and on her plate there is an apple, a salad, and vegetables. This illustration communicates volumes. One lady has a poor diet; the other lady has a good diet. The first lady's diet is high in fat and sugar; the second lady has a diet made up of wholesome foods. The first lady looks anxious, suspicious, irritable, and ill-tempered. At the bottom of the picture, under the second lady, the caption reads, "She's relaxed and confident; she's compatible and happy." Watson concluded by saying, "A diet low in whole grains but high in fat and sugar influences thought patterns negatively." What we eat does affect how we think!

Dr. Ray Williams of the Mayo Clinic in Rochester, Minnesota, did pioneer studies in the 1940s on diet and behavior. He took thiamine out of the diet of 11 women who worked together at the Mayo Clinic. He discovered a definite relationship between negative behavior and a lack of thiamine in the diet. This lack produced irritability, nervousness, and depression.

Writing almost one hundred years ago, Ellen White, an American pioneer in healthful eating, stated: "Anything that lessens physical strength enfeebles the mind and makes it less capable of discriminating between right and wrong. We become less capable of choosing the good, and have less strength of will to do that which we know to be right." *Counsels on Diet and Foods,* p. 49.

As you continue to discover the essential principles of healthful eating and put these principles into practice in your life, you will quickly begin to notice the benefits. Your health will improve. You energy level will increase. Your thinking will become clearer. You will feel more alert and positive about life.

Eating a nutritious, tasty, natural diet will produce both a healthy mind and body. Truly the ancient Scriptures are right when they declare: "Happy (fortunate) are you, O land, when your king is of a noble character and your princes eat for strength and not for drunkenness." Ecclesiastes 10:17. Eating for strength and not for mere gratification of appetite produces *physical health* and *mental joy*.

We'll continue to include additional basic principles which will not only transform your eating but will revolutionize your way of thinking, enabling you to become a more contented, self-controlled and cheerful person. Jesus said, "I am the bread of life." John 6:48. Good whole grain homemade bread satisfies the nutritional needs of the body, just as Jesus satisfies our inner spiritual needs.

Chapter

2

The King, the Prince, and the Pauper

Would you like to increase your life expectancy by as much as eleven years? What price would you pay for eleven more happy, healthy years? "Impossible," you say. "When the finger of fate points to my end, my time is up." In the ancient Hindu philosophy, millions of people believe that very concept. They have the strange notion that when the finger of fate points to them, their life is over.

In our previous chapter we discovered that health is not a matter of chance. It's a matter of obedience to nature's laws. We can either violate nature's laws and predispose ourselves to premature death, or obey nature's laws and add years of happiness to our lives. If a formula for longevity could be put into a pill, would you take it? Of course you would.

After conducting extensive research, Dr. Lester Breslow, Dean of the School of Health at the University of California at Los Angeles, made a startling assertion: "It is possible, by following seven basic health guidelines, to increase American life expectancy by eleven years."

Let's look at these seven principles. First, Dr. Breslow suggested, avoid tobacco. Second, limit the use of alcohol. Many researchers feel we would do well to eliminate alcohol altogether. Third, avoid eating between meals. Fourth, get adequate rest (seven to eight hours per night). Fifth, engage in frequent exercise. Sixth, remain close to your ideal weight. Seventh, eat a good breakfast every day.

Here are seven vital principles of health. And this is certainly something that is achievable, something that is do-able. Breslow knew that as well. The violation of as few as two of these principles on a regular, consistent basis limits life expectancy.

Let's focus on the last of these basic seven health principles — eating a good breakfast. An old but wise saying goes, "Eat breakfast like a king, lunch like a prince, and supper like a pauper." Many people feel too rushed or too tired to eat a good breakfast. They may not sense the importance of breakfast, so they skip it. This occurs particularly when they are up late at night and have eaten a late, heavy meal. When they awaken they aren't hungry; they have no desire to eat a good breakfast. Others feel they want to lose weight and skipping breakfast is a good way to do it.

Statistics indicate that only one in 20 children have a substantial breakfast. Among the teenage group 48% of the girls and 24% of the boys don't eat breakfast at all.

"So what?" somebody asks. Does it really make any difference? What do these statistics reveal? Is there a relationship between a poor quality breakfast and mental attitudes? Does the typical breakfast of highly-refined cereals, coffee, and donuts contribute to the western world's growing epidemic of heart disease and cancer? What are the advantages of a substantial breakfast? What composes a nutritionally sound morning meal? In this chapter we'll explore answers to these vital questions.

Benefits of a Substantial Breakfast

One of the classic reports on the benefits of a good breakfast is entitled the "Iowa Breakfast Studies." A number of years ago, the United States Government studied thousands of children in the state of Iowa in an attempt to evaluate whether eating a good breakfast made any difference in their classroom attitudes, their ability to learn, and their all-around performance. These massive studies indicated the detrimental effect of skipping breakfast and the positive benefits of eating a good breakfast. In a pilot program conducted by the U.S. Department of Agriculture on 12- to 14-year-old boys, the results were astounding. The studies indicated that among the detrimental effects of skipping breakfast were a lowered attention span as well as poorer classroom attitudes. Those students who skipped breakfast tended to be much more fidgety and anxious; they were prone to be significantly more restless, and their general attitudes and thoughts tended to be much poorer.

Among the beneficial effects of eating a good breakfast are: increased attention span, positive classroom attitudes, and a greater learning ability (memory). Let's suppose that two students are seated side by side in the old city grammar school. Jimmy's mother hasn't read *Lifestyle 2000* and when he awakens in the morning he just has cold milk and a sugar-laden donut to eat. But Johnny's mom has read *Lifestyle 2000* from cover to cover! When Johnny awakens in the morning, he eats nutritious, wholesome orange slices, whole wheat toast, and a generous bowl of hot cereal.

Jimmy, who has eaten only the donut and milk, wakes up in the morning tired, somewhat grumpy. Why? Because he went to bed at 11:00 the night before after eating pizza at 10:30. Johnny, on the other hand, gets up filled with zest and eagerness to face the day, because he went to bed at 9:00, having eaten his last meal around 5:30.

As Jimmy and Johnny enter the classroom, one enters with a negative attitude and the other with a positive attitude. About mid-morning, Jimmy's blood sugar begins to sag; he's tired, yawning. Not only has he had a rough night, but coupled with a lack of nutrients in the morning, he's not prepared for the day's challenges and activities. So by mid-morning, exhausted, he puts his head on the desk. Johnny, however, is bright; his mind is alert and sharp. One boy ends up with a C-, the other boy an A. What's the difference? Lifestyle practices.

In fact, Harvard nutritionist, Dr. John Monet, said that some brands of cereal should be considered candy. He pointed out that many of the cereals on the market today have anywhere from a 25% to a 50% sugar content. He also pointed out that the lack of a good breakfast contributes to poor attitudes and possibly lower grades in students. It has been demonstrated that workers who eat a good breakfast have a better attitude toward their work and much greater efficiency on the job. Their work loss time is significantly less, and the spoilage in their work is less than people who eat no breakfast or a poor quality breakfast.

Do you have trouble sleeping? Are there some nights when you toss and turn? A good breakfast can help regulate the circadian rhythms, or sleep patterns, in the body. These sleep patterns, are unbalanced in people who regularly skip breakfast, which then leads to eating late at night. Once one eats late at night, the food must be digested. Your body attempts to rest, but the digestive system must work.

Consequently, there is a tossing and turning all night. Maybe you remember eating that great Italian meal just before going to bed — spaghetti, meatballs, salad, pasta, Italian bread, apple pie for dessert, and ice cream for more dessert. Did you ever eat anything like that at 9:30 or 10:00 at night? If you did, it's likely you had a poor night's sleep, spinning like a top. Eating late at night just doesn't work well.

A good breakfast also provides essential vitamins and minerals, enabling the body to function at peak energy levels throughout the morning, thus reducing the typical mid-morning tiredness and the need for coffee. Coffee, of course, contains an artificial stimulant, caffeine, that jolts the nervous system without providing adequate nutrients and vitamins. Coffee has been associated with such things as irritability, nervousness, anxiety, and muscle tremors. Dr. Olgsby Paul of Northwestern University has associated even moderate coffee drinking with a rise in heart disease. American women have skyrocketing bladder cancer rates. One of the reasons, researchers indicated, is because of excessive coffee drinking.

So — if you desire to have positive mental attitudes, greater memory, longer attention spans, and an overall positive learning attitude, and you want your children to have the same, if you desire to have greater efficiency at work, start out by eating a good breakfast.

Dietary Fiber and Your Health

Modern medical researchers have concluded that dietary fiber aids in reducing the risk of both heart disease and cancer. We introduced the value of fiber in the diet when discussing the value of homemade bread. You'll remember that dietary fiber is essential to good health. It's found in fresh fruits, whole grain, bran, beans, vegetables — especially carrots, and other natural products. It is what remains from plant material that can't be digested by the enzymes of our gastro-intestinal tract, largely cellulose and related substances.

One of the men who has done the pioneer research in the area of fiber is Dr. Denis Burkitt in England. He has published his conclusions in a number of medical journals, beginning in the early to mid 1970s. Dr. Burkitt pointed out that fiber helps to reduce the transit time of harmful waste materials in the intestines and bowels. This reduced transit time lessens the time of contact, thus reducing the possibility of bowel cancer. Those countries where the people's diet produces slow transit times have high cancer rates. Those countries where the diet is higher in fiber, thus producing a shorter transit time, have lowered bowel cancer rates.

Bowel cancer is growing rapidly in western society. It is a major concern among cancer specialists and researchers. Evidently a diet that is highly refined does not have sufficient bulk to move waste materials through the bowel, whereas a diet that is high in fiber has that added bulk, and moves those materials through the bowel rapidly. For example, Dr. Burkitt pointed out that the transit time of the Bantu native averages 34 hours. That is the time for the food that he has eaten to be fully digested, the waste materials to be deposited in the bowel and then to be eliminated by the body. The transit time of the average Englishman is from 80 to 120 hours. There are waste materials from food still in the bowels four days after it has been eaten!

The Bantu diet is largely grain. It is very coarse, and high in roughage. The English diet is more highly refined. There is a lot more fat and sugar. In every society in the world where there is a highly refined diet consisting largely of sugars and fats, the bowel cancer rate is unusually high. In those societies where the diet is high in fiber, the bowel cancer rate is low. One of the best reasons to eat a good, healthy breakfast is to prevent this type of degenerative disease brought on by wrong choices in dietary habits. One of the ways to reduce the bowel cancer rate is to have a diet high in fiber.

A high-fiber diet has another benefit. Evidently cholesterol in the body attaches to fiber molecules. The waste materials (fecal matter) of those individuals in societies where dietary fiber is high contain higher amounts of cholesterol. Interestingly enough, individuals who have eaten a diet high in fiber have less problems with blockage of coronary arteries. A high-fiber diet, therefore, reduces the risk of both coronary heart disease and cancer. It improves attitudes, increases daily efficiency, and maximizes the possibility of success. These are certainly good reasons to get up a little earlier to prepare a good wholesome breakfast for your family.

Cereals, Eggs and Bacon

Be careful, though, of cereals which are high in sugar. You remember that Dr. Monet of Harvard University said some cereals should be called candy! Dr. Ira Shannon and his co-workers at the Veterans Administration Hospital in Houston, Texas, analyzed 78 ready-to-eat breakfast cereals for their overall sugar content. To their amazement, they discovered that 23 of the cereals proved to be 20% to 25% sugar, while 24 of the 78 were a whopping 25% to 40% sugar.

Whole grain cereals provide protein, calcium, iron, trace minerals, B-vitamins, vitamin E in the germ and, of course, fiber in the bran.

You may be wondering, "What about the traditional breakfast of bacon, eggs, and coffee?" Dr. C. Bruce Taylor, professor of Pathology at Northwestern University Medical School, as reported in the *Washington Star*, declared: "The best way for a woman to kill her husband is to feed him one egg per day." Now, I'm sure none of my friends reading this book want to murder their husbands. Yet by giving him two or three eggs every morning for six months, your spouse's cholesterol level could go so high that he could die of a heart attack. We could call this, "Murder at the Breakfast Table." You won't even be found out. I say this with tongue-in-cheek, but it is very serious business.

Dr. Taylor says that the yolk of an egg contains about all the cholesterol the human body can handle in one day without developing fatty patches in the heart and brain arteries over the years. Dr. Taylor is an authority on the effects of diet and arteriosclerosis. Many hospital Health Education Departments encourage their patients to eat no more than three eggs per week. This, of course, is in harmony with the recommendations of the American Medical Association.

You may be wondering, does this include those eggs you would use in cooking? The answer is yes. The age-old daily breakfast of bacon and eggs, consisting of enormous levels of high fat, is becoming a thing of the past. In fact, eliminating eggs from the diet entirely is the best of all. Close to 60% of all deaths in the United States come from coronary heart disease or related heart problems. If we are going to reverse this trend, it necessitates revolutionary changes in our diet, moving away from high-fat choices to a diet high in fiber; from one high in refined foods to one high in natural foods. This is another reason to prepare your own delicious, delightful breakfast dishes, especially breakfast cereals.

Breakfast and Digestion

You know, when you get up in the morning, it usually has been between eight to 12 hours since your last meal. Your glucose or blood sugar level is at its lowest point in the day. Glucose is the basic fuel for the brain and central nervous system. A good breakfast will keep you from being tired and irritable by mid-morning. Since the stomach is rested, these are two real advantages of eating a large, healthy, nutritious breakfast.

By morning, the bulk of the digestion process is over. All previous meals are well digested and the stomach is ready to receive more food. The stomach has rested during the night. Digestion has come to a halt, as well as those body functions that are not needed.

Digestive juices have been secreted by the stomach upon awakening to prepare for the thorough digestion of your food. These bodies of ours are an amazing, carefully engineered workmanship. They give evidence, not of chance or happenstance or accident, but of design in creation. It has been amazing for me to recognize that approximately an hour before breakfast, the stomach begins to secrete digestive juices to prepare for the morning meal. The body goes into action, hoping and longing for a good breakfast. It is for that reason that breakfast eaten on an empty stomach can be easily digested, and the vitamins and minerals quickly assimilated into the bloodstream.

Guidelines for a Good Breakfast

What are the guidelines for a good breakfast? Remember the old saying, "Eat breakfast like a king, lunch like a prince, and supper like a pauper." A good breakfast should be:

1. Nutritious — supplying at least one third to one half of the day's food needs. It should include:
   - one serving of either cooked or fresh fruit
   - one serving of whole grains with some form of milk (either cold or hot; or possibly waffles, pancakes, etc.)
   - one to two slices of whole grain bread

The milk can be soy milk, nut milk, or you may desire to use cow's milk. We suggest the gradual elimination of all animal products from the diet, since animal products tend to be more disease prone. First, eliminate meats that are extremely high in fats, such as pork and marbled steaks. Then reduce lean meats, finally cutting them out altogether. Then limit the number of eggs you eat and the cheeses in your diet and move toward a diet of fruits, nuts, grains, and vegetables.

All dietary change, of course, must be gradual. So, we suggest that you begin these changes, not radically, but by gradually substituting dishes that your family enjoys in the diet. But let's go back to those guidelines for a good breakfast. It should be:

2. Appetizing and attractive. If the table is set in a very attractive way, most of the family will be much more prone to eat a good breakfast early in the morning.

To avoid being rushed in the morning, often in our home I would set the table the night before so the children would be attracted and enticed by breakfast. One evening

I set the table around 10:00. It was beautifully laid out, with bowls for cereal and plates for fruit and toast, and a nice tablecloth. We had some friends drop in unexpectedly at 10:30 at night, and they talked until about 11:00 or 11:15. The friends looked at me and said, "My, you folk really eat late suppers around here. What time do you eat — 11:00 or 11:30?" I then explained I was setting the table for breakfast. Although people may misunderstand if you set the table late at night, it certainly is worth it in the morning and might save you some time, too. Keep breakfast:

3. Unhurried. If the breakfast is ready on time, allowing adequate time to eat, and individuals don't have to rush, they will eat more and better.
4. Simple and easy to eat — not having large varieties of food.
5. A family meal. It is a very special feeling of bonding to start the day together at breakfast time.

Upon awakening in the morning, why not try this simple routine? Begin your day by thanking God for another day of life. Spend a little time thinking about Him. Read a verse from the Bible, maybe from the book of Psalms. Set your mind in a peaceful attitude. Drink a couple glasses of water. Take a 15-minute walk, then eat a good breakfast.

Although this may require getting up a little sooner (maybe thirty minutes earlier), the rewards of good health, a positive mental attitude, and a closer walk with God will be well worth it. So try starting your day with a little spiritual fellowship with God, some exercise, and a great breakfast. This physical, mental, and spiritual approach will provide you with the strength and courage necessary to face whatever problems may come your way that day.

Planning a Balanced Menu

We are now going to focus specifically on low-fat, low-cholesterol foods that taste great and will help us reduce the risk of a heart attack. Are you aware of the fact that one in every four American men will suffer a heart attack before the age of 60? That's pretty sobering, isn't it? If I began to count, and every time I came to the number four I placed my finger on you in this reading "audience," either you (if you're male) or your husband (if you are female) would have a heart attack before the age of 60.

Yet the evidence is mounting! Heart disease, America's number-one killer, can often be prevented, and diet plays a significant role in reducing our risk of death from a heart attack. Myron Coenick, Director of the Institute of Human Nutrition at Columbia University, stated: "The evidence for a relationship between fat and cholesterol and coronary artery disease, cancer and diabetes has become so solid that only the most diehard would deny it." Medical researchers throughout the world agree that our high-fat diet contributes to a high incidence of heart disease.

The American diet is approximately 40% fat. The Senate Select Subcommittee on Nutrition recommended that Americans reduce the fat in their diet by at least 10% to have a maximum of 30% of the diet that is made up of fat. Today, that figure is considered still too high by many. They also recommended that cholesterol intake be reduced to 300 mg per day. There are times that these figures stagger us and we wonder whether or not we have to weigh out every gram of fat we eat. Obviously not.

In this book, we want to represent a natural lifestyle that includes large amounts of fruits, nuts, grains, and vegetables. If you choose from a wide variety of natural foods, you need not be overly concerned about excessive fat. To illustrate how little 300 mg a day is, one egg contains a whopping 250 mg of fat. Any diet designed to reduce fat in the diet must drastically reduce the amount of animal products.

Well, you ask, if I reduce the amount of animal products in my diet, what am I going to eat? Where will I get adequate protein? Does this mean that I must become a so-called "grass eater," as some people call vegetarians? Let's discover a few facts about cholesterol, and then look at the abundance of all the good things we can eat besides high-fat foods.

Cholesterol Facts

Cholesterol is a fatty substance manufactured by the body. It is also present in all foods of animal origin. Vegetable products do not contain cholesterol. Some contain limited amounts of fat which the body may use to produce cholesterol, but only animal products contain cholesterol which is ingested directly. Therefore, if you're going to work on reducing the amount of cholesterol in the diet, it's necessary to reduce not only the amount of animal products, but all fat and oil in the diet, and to increase the amount of natural food products.

Why is cholesterol harmful to the body, and how does it affect it? Most cholesterol enters the blood and is carried around in packets called lipoproteins. These microscopic-sized particles are made up largely of fat, cholesterol, and protein. They act like trucks. If you look at the diagram below, the lipoproteins are containers that carry cholesterol.

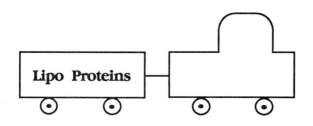

Trucking Cholesterol Away
From Local Scene

Now, there's a problem when cholesterol is not trucked away. It becomes deposited on the arterial walls, leading to hardening of the arteries and coronary heart disease. The more of this cholesterol that remains on the arterial walls, the more obstructed the artery becomes.

Notice the following diagrams. On the left you have an unobstructed artery, on the right, one that is partially obstructed, and then the artery in the bottom center that is almost totally blocked off.

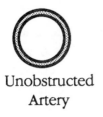
Unobstructed
Artery

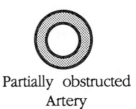
Partially obstructed
Artery

Blocked off
Artery

When arteries become blocked off like this one, free-flowing fat in the bloodstream acts like a plug or clog and inhibits blood flow. As a result, the heart squeezes and pumps, but being unable to pump blood through the blocked arteries, suffers spasm, heart attack, oxygen deprivation, and ultimately death.

You can see that it's absolutely imperative to keep our arteries open and free from clogging in order to maintain good health. Of course, this is another reason why a diet low in cholesterol, combined with a good exercise program, keeps one in optimum health. You will remember exercise, as well as diet, is one of Dr. Braslow's health laws in the previous chapter.

As we have already mentioned, one of the big problems in diet is fat. Let's look at some practical facts regarding fat and how you can keep your arteries unobstructed. There are two kinds of fats: polyunsaturated and saturated. Polyunsaturated fats are fats of vegetable origin. Most of the time these are liquid at room temperature. Although some vegetable fats may be hardened at room temperature, placing them in the saturated fats category, usually saturated fats are of animal origin. These hard fats are mostly solid at room temperature and tend to elevate blood cholesterol.

One way to reduce your cholesterol is to use less saturated fats and replace them with polyunsaturated fats. So, rather than using meat fats, shortening, butter, cream, whole milk and egg yolk, you would rather choose far lesser amounts of sunflower oil, corn oil, soy oil, cottonseed oil, or any products containing vegetable oil, soy milk, or nut milks. You might want to use egg replacers rather than egg yolk, and rather than chocolate, which tends to be high in fat, use carob. The chart below is a good guide.

Use little or no saturated fats	Use a minimal amount of polyunsaturated fats
Meat fats	Sunflower oil
Shortening	Corn oil
Butter	Soy oil
Cream	Cottonseed oil
Whole Milk	Any products containing vegetable oils: soy milk, nut milks
Egg yolk	Egg replacers
Chocolate	Carob

If you are predominantly eating the items listed on the left side of the chart, your cholesterol level will tend to be high. If you are eating minimally of items found on the right of the chart, your cholesterol level should become significantly lower. Should you have a major problem with coronary artery disease, then you should eliminate visible fats from your diet altogether, or dramatically reduce them.

Even polyunsaturated fats should not be used in abundance, since the body uses them and then manufactures cholesterol. The more "natural" the diet, the less one has to be concerned with fats.

Relationship Between Diet and Heart Disease

As mentioned earlier, recent studies have evaluated the fat content in the diet of a nation and then compared this fat content to the rate at which the people are dying from coronary heart disease. The results are similar worldwide. This similarity — despite cultural differences, genetic variants, and changing environments — is truly remarkable. The simple principle is: If the people in the nation have a diet traditionally high in saturated fats, they also have an extremely high rate of coronary heart disease.

Some of the leading heart attack rates in Europe are in Finland. The Finns, due to their extremely northern latitude, eat lesser amounts of fresh fruits, nuts, grains, and vegetables than do the Greeks, who are in a much more temperate climate. The Finns eat a diet high in meat and animal fats. The Greeks, on the other hand, eat more fresh fruits and a lot more of the natural, polyunsaturated fats, like olive oil. Result? Finns have extremely high heart attack rates, while the Greeks have much lower rates.

Some studies were done not long ago at one of the Finnish mental hospitals. The Finnish cardiologist took two groups of individuals. One group was given skim milk, vegetable oil, soft margarine, and a low-fat diet. The other group received whole milk, animal fats, butter, and the average Finnish high-fat diet. At the end of six years, death rates from coronary heart disease were twice as high in the group on a high-fat diet. The groups were then switched for six more years. The results: The situation reversed itself when the two groups switched diets. Once again, here is a remarkable indication that our high-fat diet leads to heart disease.

In Los Angeles, the Veterans Administration Hospital was the site of a massive study on coronary heart disease. The veterans were split into two groups with each being assigned a different cafeteria. In one, polyunsaturated fats were used instead of saturated animal fats. In the other the normal high-fat American diet was served. At the end of eight years the group on the high-fat diet suffered a dramatic increase in heart attacks.

One of the classic studies in North America on heart disease occurred as well in California, among fifty thousand Seventh-day Adventists. Since Seventh-day Adventists don't smoke, their known cancer rates have been markedly less. This team of researchers wanted to evaluate not only cancer, but heart disease. These fifty thousand Seventh-day Adventists completed extremely thorough health questionnaires. Their personal medical records were carefully examined, their dietary principles were closely evaluated, the amount of fat in their diet was scrutinized. The health statistics of these Adventists were then compared to the general California population. Vegetarian Adventist men, carefully following a low-fat dietary regime and on an overall balanced lifestyle program, had an overwhelming advantage. The studies revealed that the Adventist men lived seven years longer than their non-Adventist counterparts.

Also discovered was an advantage of eight to one in reducing heart attacks. A non-Adventist in the study was eight times as likely to suffer such an attack. Certainly the Adventists have an advantage. But by dramatically reducing the fat in your diet and making significant lifestyle changes, you can have the same advantage the Adventists have.

Evaluating Your Personal Risk of Heart Attack

Now, of course, coronary heart disease has other contributing risk factors besides a high-fat diet. Medical researchers usually recognize that no one factor causes a heart attack. Most list approximately ten risk factors contributing to a heart attack. Let's review these major risk factors. As we do, place a check in the box beside any risk factor which applies to you in the chart on the following page. The more checks you have, the more likely you are to be predisposed to a heart attack. The fewer checks you have, the less likely you are to have a heart attack. Now, don't have a heart attack because you have too many checks in the boxes! Just be aware that there is something you can do about eight of the 10 of these boxes.

Risk Factor	Place Check Here
1. Male	❏
2. Hereditary factors (it runs in the family)	❏
3. Little physical activity (no organized exercise program)	❏
4. Inner stress	❏
5. Elevated blood cholesterol (over 200 mg)	❏
6. High blood pressure	❏
7. Overweight (more than 10 lbs.)	❏
8. Cigarette smoking	❏
9. Coffee drinking (more than three cups per day)	❏
10. Insufficient sleep (less than six hrs. per night consistently)	❏

Number one, are you a *male*? Men seem to have a greater predisposition to heart disease than women. Women have some built-in factors before menopause that help to reduce the cholesterol on a monthly basis. After menopause in women, the chances of a coronary even out.

Number two, *hereditary factors*. Does heart disease run in your family? Do you have a father, mother, sister, or brother — someone in the immediate family — who has had a heart attack? If you do, check number 2.

Three, *little physical activity*. Chasing the children around the house all day, or walking from the car to the office many times a day because you're a traveling salesman don't count. If you do not have a planned exercise program in which you're exercising vigorously for 30 minutes at least four times a week, you should check number 3.

There are two kinds of exercise programs here that are okay. Engage in some activity that causes you to sweat — racquetball, jogging, cycling, or swimming, three to four times a week. Walking for half an hour in the morning and evening is a great way to exercise. But if you do not have organized physical activity, you should check box number 3. Now there *is* an exception for people who may have an extremely intense job where they get an abundant amount of active physical exercise.

Number four, *stress*. Are you the kind of person who is laid back, who will let things go? Do you have the inner attitude that everything's going to be all right? Or are you quite aggressive, quite pushy, striving constantly to get ahead? Are you able to sit down and relax or do you have a difficult time relaxing? Are you a Type A personality (more aggressive) or a Type B person (more naturally relaxed)?

You can evaluate whether you seem to be motivated by inner stress — anxiety, worry, tension, in a rush, constantly pushing. Do you let other people finish their sentences or do you jump in before they do? Are you a person who is quick to react? If you feel you are motivated by inner stress, check this.

Point five, *blood cholesterol.* If your diet is high in fat, and your cholesterol is over 200, you should check number four. If you eat a predominantly vegetarian diet, you may not need to check that point.

Number six, *high blood pressure.* Average blood pressure is 120/80. Has your doctor told you that you have high blood pressure?

Number seven, *overweight.* Are you more than 10 pounds overweight? If you wonder here, strip to the waist, stand sideways in front of a mirror. If there is quite a midriff bulge, you're probably more than 10 pounds too heavy. Somebody said if you can pinch an inch, it's too much.

Point eight, *cigarette smoking.* If you smoke, check box number 8. Cigarette smoking has been directly linked to increased heart disease.

Number nine, *coffee drinking.* Dr. Olgsby Paul has pointed out that if you drink any more than three cups a day, it may predispose you to a coronary heart attack. Of course, even moderate amounts of coffee can cause irritability. For heart disease, if you're drinking more than three cups a day, you should check number nine.

Number ten, *insufficient sleep.* Insufficient sleep is also a contributor to coronary heart disease. If you get less than six hours of sleep per night, check this box.

Now add up your score. How many boxes have you checked? As few as two risk factors indicate the need of dietary control. Three or four risk factors indicate a good possibility of a heart attack, while over five necessitate immediate attention. "Why," you say, "I wish you wouldn't have told me that. I felt quite good before I picked up this book. Now I feel so anxious, I may have a heart attack right here."

It is interesting to note that six of the ten risk factors have some relationship to diet. Here is the good news. Look down your list again. You can't do anything if you are a male; you can't do anything about heredity. But you can do something about the eight others. Let's pause for a moment to think about the heart attack risk factors which are in some ways related to diet.

First, *little physical activity* might be related to our diet. Often people are overweight, so they don't want to exercise.

Inner stress. Many people have a high-sugar diet, and one low in vitamin B. Therefore, their ability to manage the daily stresses is diminished. In addition to exercise, diet can help you in this area.

Elevated blood cholesterol is certainly related to diet. High blood pressure may be related to diet, since excessive salt in the diet contributes to it. Being *overweight* is definitely related to diet. Often people gain weight because they eat large amounts of food between meals.

Cigarette smoking may also be related to diet. Individuals with a highly spiced diet will have a much more difficult time giving up cigarette smoking. *Coffee drinking*, of course, is diet-related. A significant number of these points have to do with what one consumes.

The good news is that it is possible to do something about eight of the above 10 risk factors. We can make choices to change faulty lifestyle habit patterns into positive, health-building ones.

You know, we are not simply enlarged protein molecules! We're certainly not genetic animals that can't make moral choices. One of the key factors in any change is a recognition that you can alter the course of your life. Let's recognize that we are not pre-programmed to failure; deep within the fabric of our thinking, in the core of our being, an all-loving Creator has given us the ability to make rational choices. When we choose to bring our lifestyle practices into harmony with the laws of our being, radical changes will take place.

Let me give you some practical hints on how to control cholesterol. Since dietary fat (amount and type) is directly related to coronary heart disease, a blood cholesterol of over 250 mg presents four times the risk of a heart attack than one less than 200 mg. The following practical steps will help lower the blood cholesterol:

1. Change the type of fat consumed from animal to vegetable.
2. Use nut milks, soy milk or skim milk. Limit the use of whole milk and cheeses.
3. Use eggs sparingly.
4. Lower or eliminate flesh foods or meat products.
5. Limit the use of fried foods (such as potato chips, french fries, those foods fried in heavy grease).
6. Control the intake of sugars in all forms (but particularly be careful about white, brown, and raw sugar).
7. Eat a wide variety of vegetables, fruits, nuts, and whole grains.

These seven steps will help you reduce the risk of a heart attack.

Guide To the Basic Four Food Groups

U.S. News and World Report interviewed a number of experts in nutrition and published their responses in an article entitled "Experts' Recipes for a Healthy Life," January 20, 1986. Michael Jacobson, Executive Director for the Center for Science in the Public Interest, stated: "The consensus is that Americans should be eating less fat, cholesterol, sodium (that is salt), and refined sugars and eating more starch and dietary fiber. The best foods for you are beans, grains, fresh fruits, vegetables, and low-fat dairy, meat and poultry foods. The worst foods for you are hot dogs, fatty steaks, cheeseburgers, fried foods, soda pop, most pastries, and ice cream." Although we personally question the value of using any meat at all, we certainly believe that if we choose from the first list, beans, grains, fresh fruits and vegetables, and try to eliminate the last list, we'll be doing much, much better.

Vegetarianism is not some out-moded, weird, strange, bizarre, kooky, extreme, faddist diet! Walter Mertz, Director of the Agriculture Department, Human Nutrition Research Center, was right on target when he said, "The rule should be — everything in balance."

A balanced vegetarian diet includes a wide variety of foods from the food groups listed below: It includes at least two to three servings from the bread and cereal group (including varying types of milks). It includes three to four daily servings of cooked or raw vegetables, three to four servings of canned or fresh fruit, and two to three servings of protein. This makes a minimum of 10 servings of food a day, and a maximum of about 14. You certainly don't have to count the servings you eat. Concentrate on a wide variety of wholesome, nutritious, raw or cooked fresh fruits, nuts, grains, or vegetables.

Here is a sample of possible healthy food options for a day.

Daily Guide for a Balanced Menu

Breakfast

1 serving whole grain cereal, cooked cereal
    or other main dish

1 to 2 pieces of whole wheat toast

1 serving fresh fruit

1 serving cooked fruit (canned applesauce,
    peaches, etc.)

1 serving milk or soy milk

Dinner

1 to 2 servings carbohydrate

1 to 2 servings cooked vegetables (beans, corn,
    peas, etc.)

1 to 2 servings raw vegetables
    (salads — tossed, cabbage, carrot)

1 to 2 servings protein

optional: bread

Supper

Soups and crackers — or
fruit and toast — or
sandwiches and fruit

Remember that eighty percent of our food intake for the day should come at our first two meals. With children in school, and working, this may be a little bit difficult for many families to achieve. Supper often becomes dinner, or the evening meal. If this is true, it is best to eat your dinner or supper, that larger meal, as early in the evening as possible. Then get up and do a little exercise afterward to avoid the additional calories being generated into fat. Exercise will help to burn off those calories, and will be good for the entire system. The later you're eating the evening meal without any exercise, the more difficult sleep will become.

We have found that mealtimes of 7:30 a.m., 12:30 p.m. and 5:30 p.m. to be a good eating schedule. It gives your system five hours before the next meal to assimilate and digest your food. It also enables you to have adequate exercise before retiring. If your food is digested before going to sleep, your stomach will not have to labor all night.

As you look over this balanced guide for eating, you will begin to recognize that our loving Creator has given us an abundance of natural foods to sustain life and prolong health. After creating the amazing variety of fruits, nuts, grains, and vegetables, He declared: "Ye may freely eat." Genesis 2:16.

As you make wise selections from these basic four food groups, you may eat until your heart is content. Food is meant to be enjoyed. The healthier you eat, the more you'll enjoy it, and the longer you will live to continue to enjoy it.

Please look at the chart on pages 39-42. This is a cholesterol guide that will assist you in choosing low cholesterol foods. The left column indicates the category of food, the center column indicates foods recommended in that category, and the right column describes foods to avoid.

Low-Cholesterol, Low-Fat, Low-Sugar Diet

Type of Food	Foods Recommended	Foods to Avoid
Beverages (non-dairy)	Unsweetened fruit and vegetable juices, cereal beverages.	Alcohol of all kinds. Coffee, tea, and most carbonated beverages.
Fruits	Any fresh, frozen, or dried fruits or fruit juices. Canned fruits in fruit juices.	Highly sweetened fruits and juices.
Breads	Whole grain breads: whole wheat, rye, corn, and breads made with a mixture of flours.	Most commercially made white breads, cookies, cakes, and pastries.

Type of Food	Foods Recommended	Foods to Avoid
Cereals	All cooked cereals and whole grain products. Dry cereals of granola type.	Dry cereals with a high sugar content.
Fats	A minimum of all vegetable oils; soft sunflower or corn oil margarines; homemade mayonnaise; peanut butter, olives. All nuts and seeds (pumpkin, sesame, sunflower).	Butter and cream; lard; hydrogenated margarines and shortenings; bacon and meat drippings; cream sauces and gravies unless specially made with polyunsaturated fats; commercial mayonnaise.

Type of Food	Foods Recommended	Foods to Avoid
Meats	Meat substitutes made of vegetable protein may be used. Legumes such as beans, peas, lentils, and garbanzos will adequately substitute for meat.	Pork and pork products; egg yolk; all shellfish; poultry skin; all organ meats; luncheon meat products such as hot dogs and sandwich meats; regular hamburger; most frozen or packaged dinners.
Soups	Meat-free vegetable soups; soups made with soy, nut, or skim milk; lentil, bean, and pea soups.	

Type of Food	Foods Recommended	Foods to Avoid
Sweets	Fresh fruits, natural dried fruits such as raisins, dates, figs.	Cakes, candies, jams, jellies, ice cream, sodas, and shakes.
Vegetables	Any fresh, frozen, or canned (check for sugar).	Any buttered, creamed, or fried (unless in vegetable oil).

Chapter

4

The Advantages
of a Vegetarian Diet

This chapter is one of the most informative of the entire book. We'll explore the advantages of the vegetarian diet and share with you recipes that will help you find your way toward becoming a vegetarian. Don't get nervous; we're not going to take all of your meat away all at once! The principles we're going to share with you in this chapter will enable you to cut all meat out of your diet if you want. That choice, of course, is up to you. Not only will we share with you the scientific facts of the advantages of a vegetarian diet, but we'll also include a variety of healthful, nutritious, and extremely tasty vegetarian dishes.

A growing number of Americans are either limiting the amount of meat in their diet or discarding it altogether. According to a recent survey, over twelve million people in the United States claim they are vegetarians. The figures have jumped by over 400% in the last twenty-five years. Vegetarianism is steadily growing in popularity.

Contrary to popular belief, the word "vegetarian" is not derived from the word "vegetable." Many people think so, but it's just not true. The word "vegetarian" comes from the latin word "vegus" which means "whole, sound, fresh, lively." As you adopt a vegetarian diet, you're cooperating with the very laws of your being.

Vegetarianism is a wholistic approach to health, focusing on the physical, mental, and spiritual dimensions of life. What you eat affects the quality of your blood. A poor quality of food produces a corresponding poor quality of blood. This poor quality of blood, of course, affects the brain, resulting in brain functions that are not as clear. Consequently, diet plays a significant role in attitude and disposition.

This information is designed not merely to give you physical health, but to help you have a better, more joyful outlook on life, and thus a deeper understanding of the purpose of life. We were made to be in harmony with both the laws of our physical being, and our Creator, the God who made us. So the very word "vegetarian" means "whole." It has to do with wholistic health in its total aspect.

Some vegetarians exclude eating meat for moral reasons, others for ethical reasons, but many for strictly health reasons. Vegetarians don't necessarily do all their shopping at health food stores. Most shop at ordinary grocery stores and just skip the meat.

Throughout history, many of the world's brightest minds and most creative personalities have been vegetarians. George Bernard Shaw, the English playwright, could not bring himself to "eat the flesh of dead carcasses." Two of the world's longest living civilizations, the Hunzas in the Himalayas, and the Otomai Indians of South America are predominantly vegetarians. Some in these civilizations are living to be 130 to 140 years old. In fact, the late Dr. Paul Dudley White visited the Himalayas in northern Pakistan some time ago. This famous heart specialist from Boston examined Hunzas in their 90s and discovered that their veins and arteries were similar to American men in their 30s.

According to the National Academy of Science's National Research Council, which publishes the Recommended Daily Allowances for U.S. Food, "All but the most restricted vegetarian diets are nutritionally safe." This is certainly confirmed by the studies of Dr. Paul Dudley White on the Hunzas and other studies around the world. As long as vegetarians eat a wide variety of fruits, nuts, grains, and vegetables, they will normally receive adequate protein.

In this chapter, you will discover how to prepare delicious low-cholesterol, vegetarian protein dishes. You may have wondered, "Does the vegetarian diet provide adequate protein? What advantages does a vegetarian diet have over a meat diet? Is vegetable protein complete? Does it really matter if a protein source is complete or not? How much protein does one really need?" You will find the answers to these questions.

Fundamental Facts About Protein

There are many misconceptions about protein today. Some people think that if you don't eat meat, you won't get adequate protein.

Proteins are composed of amino acids. The body manufactures amino acids from the foods we eat. Those amino acids which cannot be produced by the body are called essential amino acids. Of the 22 known amino acids, nine cannot be produced by the body and must be present in the food we eat. These essential amino acids are all present in meat. In other words, meat is a complete source of protein. The amino acids necessary for body growth and development are present in meat. But these amino acids can also be obtained from a variety of vegetable proteins eaten in combination with grains and nuts. What we're really saying is this: You can get adequate protein from meat or you can get adequate protein from vegetarian products, natural foods, that also contain the essential amino acids.

There are some basic facts to remember about proteins. It is not the amino acid content of a single protein source that is important but that of the entire daily menu. The body cannot tell whether it is getting its protein source from meat, or whether the essential amino acids are balanced in such a way that it is getting them from two or three sources at the same meal. If a diet has adequate calories and contains a wide variety of fruits, grains, and vegetables, protein is usually adequate.

Dr. Frederick Stare, Nutritionist and Professor at Harvard University, stated in his study of protein foods, published in the *American Journal of Public Health*: "As long as this country has access to a plentiful supply of calories and a variety of whole grain cereals and legumes, it is highly unlikely that impairment of health from protein deficiency will ever occur." The danger, of course, is very strict, narrow, restricted diets, such as the Zen-macrobiotic diet, which ultimately proceeds through varying stages until one eats only rice and water. This, of course, is very dangerous to health. We're not suggesting anything like this. We suggest that you eat a wide variety of large quantities of fruits, nuts, grains, and vegetables. Not at every meal, of course, but throughout the day and the week!

Complete vegetarian protein combinations include:

- all grains and legumes
- all grains and milk products
- all legumes and seeds
- milk products and either seeds or legumes

Examples might include: Rice-bean casserole, wheat bread with baked beans, bean or pea curry on rice, corn tortillas and beans, lentil soup with bread, cereal with milk, cashew nut roast with bread, wheat-soy bread, and many others.

Standard nutrition charts indicate a woman should have between 44 and 50 grams of protein, a man 52 to 56 grams, and a child 23 to 35 grams per day. However, more recent researchers feel that 56 grams of protein is nearly twice the actual human need. Vegetarian protein in combination is complete. Animal protein is also complete.

Then, you say, why be a vegetarian if both are complete sources of protein? Vegetarians have a decreased risk of heart attack, a decreased risk of cancer, a decreased risk of communicable diseases such as salmonella, brucellosis, and trichinosis. They have greater endurance. In the world in which we live today, there is an economy of land use, and the possibility of feeding the world's starving masses is much greater when people switch to vegetarianism.

Why Be a Vegetarian?

What advantages do vegetarians have? From a health standpoint, is it worth it to markedly reduce your meat intake and eventually cut it out altogether? Besides being expensive, animal proteins have health liabilities because of the high fat and disease contents attached to them. Each year there are close to 600,000 deaths in the U.S. due to coronary artery disease. This accounts for 55% of all deaths in America. Heart disease is the number one killer in the U.S.

One important key in reducing heart attack deaths is reducing the fat in the diet. As America has become more health conscious and has reduced its fat intake in the last 15 years, deaths from heart disease have been reduced in the United States by 15% to 20%. At last we're heading in the right direction! This reduction has a direct relationship with the reduction of fat in our diets.

In Japan, Greece, and Italy where levels of blood cholesterol are low compared with the average American levels, the rate of heart disorders is lower than in the United States.

John M. Chapman, of the UCLA School of Medicine, states: "A cholesterol-lowering diet in older men has resulted in significantly reducing heart attack death rates. In every country where the fat consumption is high, heart attacks are high. In those countries where fat consumption is low, heart attack death rates are low." If you look throughout the United States at groups of people where fat consumption is high, again the heart attack rate will be high. The "Framingham Study" followed the health habits of thousands of American men for more than a quarter of a century in Framingham, Massachusetts. It indicated that those with high cholesterol levels had a much higher possibility of a heart attack than those with lower cholesterol levels. A vegetarian diet markedly reduces the risk of heart disease.

In addition, the rate of cancer on a low-fat diet is reduced. "There is overwhelming evidence that cancer is related to the environment and diet is a factor, perhaps the major environmental factor," said D.M. Hegsted, Associate Director for Research of Harvard University's Research Center.

British epidemiologist, Richard Doll, believes food is number one in accounting for 35% of all tumors. Dr. Gio B. Gori, Deputy Director of the National Institute, Division of the Causes of Cancer, believes that 30% of cancer in women and 40% of cancer in men are the result of a *poor diet.*

If you would like to reduce the risk of cancer, it would be well to eliminate or greatly reduce (in your diet):

- all visible fats; animal products
- excessive high sugar foods
- highly refined foods

A number of news journals have recently published studies entitled "The Cancer Prevention Diet." This cancer prevention diet includes whole grains — wheat, barley, oats, rye; leafy green vegetables, carrots, potatoes, beets, and corn; fresh fruits or dried fruits; nuts, including seeds and beans. If we were to have two groups of food to illustrate this point, we would have on the left side a diet high in fat, animal products, sugar, and highly refined foods. On the right side we would have a diet of whole grains, leafy green vegetables, fresh and dried fruits, nuts, seeds, beans, etc. The diet on the left side, the high-fat, high-sugar, highly refined diet, would also be high in the risk of heart disease and cancer. On the other hand, those foods which reduce the risk of cancer also reduce the risk of heart disease.

One of the other real problems, of course, with a diet that is high in meat is that there is an increased risk of animal-to-man communicable diseases: salmonellosis, brucellosis, and trichinosis. Of more than 200 communicable diseases of animals, 100 are considered infectious to man and 80 are transmitted naturally between vertebrate animals and man. Commenting on salmonellosis, a bacterial disease which causes vomiting, nausea, and diarrhea, the special issue of *Life and Health* magazine, p. 16, stated: "As long as we use animal products it is a losing battle."

Reducing the risk of cancer, heart disease, and animal-related diseases is in direct proportion to reducing the amount of animal products we use in our diet.

Sometimes we're asked, "What about pesticides? Doesn't a vegetarian diet put us at risk because of the high pesticide levels? What about the sprays on fruits and vegetables?" There are some things to be concerned about, no doubt, in pesticide levels. Yet there is something to keep in mind. Meat contains concentrated pesticide levels. Meat contains 14 times more pesticides than vegetable foods (Kay S. Nelson, M.P.H., paper entitled *Vegetarianism*, p. 1).

You may be wondering, "Can I eat anything today? Is there any food that is absolutely safe, absolutely free from contamination? The air we breathe, the water we drink, and the food we eat are all somewhat tainted and polluted." In a sense, that's true. What we're attempting to do is to eat as intelligently and healthfully as possible, reducing the risk of heart disease, cancer, and a variety of other diseases. There is no way to eliminate the risk altogether, but we can significantly and markedly reduce it.

In fact, the only diet that was absolutely perfectly healthy is the diet that God gave in the Garden of Eden. The air was unpolluted then; the water, fruits, nuts, grains, and vegetables were unpolluted then, too. That was the perfect diet. Our goal is to get back as close as possible to the original diet that our loving Creator gave to man. The closer we stay to that Eden diet, the healthier we'll be. The One who made us certainly knows and understands how to keep our bodies in ideal health.

Truth About Vegetarians

Some people have the idea that a vegetarian diet leaves a person weak, emaciated, and lacking vital energy. It's obvious that the ideal diet should not only reduce the risk of disease but give us the greatest "go power" possible. We want a diet that doesn't leave us listless, lacking drive, energy and vitality to accomplish the tasks of the day.

Per-Olaf Astrand, M.D., a Swedish physician, studied a cross segment of the Swedish population to determine the best diet for athletes. The Swedes are known for their downhill and cross-country skiing. As a result, they need athletes to have the greatest possibility for endurance. In the study, athletes were given a bicycle endurance test to discover their maximum exercise time. Initially they put the group of athletes on a meat and protein diet, and discovered that endurance for vigorous exercise was approximately 60 minutes. Then these athletes were put on a mixed fuel diet (protein and carbohydrates). Their exercise time was approximately 120 minutes. Then the diet was changed to a vegetarian diet. To the researchers' surprise, the athletes' continuous exercise time rose to 180 minutes! The group on the vegetarian diet lasted nearly three times longer than those on the meat diet. This fact has been demonstrated repeatedly. Since a vegetarian diet is easier to digest, and more quickly assimilated into the bloodstream, the body is less taxed. The result? Greater vitality, greater energy, greater get-up-and-go. If you want to have that fervor for life and health, the vegetarian diet is the one for you.

Many people are concerned about another aspect of life — the high level of poverty in the world. Consider this. Two thirds of all the human population do not have enough to eat. Famine rages throughout Africa. A terrible situation of hunger exists in parts of India, China and Pakistan.

With this in mind, we raise the questions, "How can we balance the ecosystem and improve its use to feed the teeming multitudes of the world's population? Are we squandering our resources? Are we destroying our planet?" Let's see.

1. An acre of land planted in soybeans can produce 10 times as much protein as animals grazing on the same land.

2. A pound of beef costs four times as much to produce as a pound of non-flesh protein.

3. According to one estimate, feed raised on one acre of land and converted into beef will fill the protein needs of a single person for 77 days. But soybeans raised on the same acre can fill his needs for 6.1 years.

Isn't it wise for nations to shift their production from animal products to soy protein and to vegetable products? This improves the land, reduces disease, and increases the possibility for health, life, and longevity. Vegetarianism is really the way of the future for feeding the masses of the world. It's difficult to transport cattle from one country to another, but you can transport tons of grain and soybeans quite easily. This is why many thinking people, like yourselves, are leaning toward vegetarianism.

How To Become a Vegetarian

"Well," you ask, "should I throw all my meat out at once? Should I go home and take out my steaks and lamb and pork chops and throw them away this minute?" Let me give you some common-sense tips to becoming a vegetarian. We certainly don't want you to rush into something ill-informed, or ill-prepared, that would upset your family. If you begin taking away from your family, particularly your children, the food they have become accustomed to eating, this will produce extreme defensiveness! It may even produce defensiveness in your spouse. How would you feel if people started taking something away from you? Here are some common sense principles that will help you to move toward a vegetarian diet.

1. Cut "empty" calories (sugars and visible fats) at least in half. Reduce the amount of butter that you put on your bread; reduce the amount of sugar you have for dessert. Rather than having ice cream regularly, why not try some delicious fruit desserts?

2. Increase your intake of all four basic food groups. "Beef up" your intake of fruits, nuts, grains, and vegetables.

3. Experiment with a wide selection of vegetarian protein dishes until you discover a few your family really enjoys. Beginning on page 69, you will discover that we've given a significant number of vegetarian recipes. You'll have a dozen recipes there, and there are many other vegetarian cookbooks that will be able to give you additional recipes. We encourage you to begin experimenting with those to find the ones your family enjoys.

4. Substitute these tasty, nutritious vegetarian dishes for your normal meat dishes at least twice a week.

5. During a transition period, meat analogs from companies like Worthington Foods, Morning Star Farms, Cedar Lake Foods and others may be helpful. You can find these products in health food stores and in the frozen foods section in some markets. These analogs are protein substitutes that have a comparable taste to some meat products. Don't expect them to taste exactly like meat; they won't. But you can appreciate them for the uniqueness of their taste. There are vegetarian hot dogs, hamburgers, steaks, chops — and they are excellent substitutes! Our family uses them occasionally.

6. When making the change, begin by cutting out the meat high in saturated fats such as pork, marbled steaks, hamburgers, hot dogs, etc. Try to move into your new diet using primarily fish and chicken. Then, of course, remove them as well.

7. Since lifestyle change is best achieved gradually, give yourself a period of three to six months to make the complete transition.

8. Your taste buds will begin to adapt as you develop a new taste for wholesome foods such as nut roasts, peas, beans, lentils, barley, soya-protein and gluten meat substitutes.

The vegetarian diet is not new. It isn't some fad that has just sprung up on the crest of last week's health wave. The vegetarian diet dates back to the Garden of Eden. It was God's original diet for the human race. This world needs a little more of the Eden life! In Eden, human beings were whole. They were physically healthy, they were mentally happy, and they were in harmony with the God who made them. They lived a life of inner peace, physical well-being, and a closeness with our Creator. In the hectic pace of 20th century living, the diet from nature's pantry will strengthen both our minds and bodies.

You will notice on the following page that we have listed the protein content of several foods. So if you have doubts about how much protein a particular food item has, you may look it up on this very simple chart.

Protein Content of Common Foods

Food Item	Amount	Protein Amount
Whole Wheat Flour	1 c.	8-10 gm
White Flour	1/2 c.	6-10 gm
Brewer's Yeast	1/2 c.	50 gm
Eggs	1	6 gm
Milk	1 c.	8 gm
Skim Milk	7/8 c.	7 gm
Soy Milk	7/8 c.	7 gm
Cottage Cheese	1/2 c.	20 gm
Soy Beans	1/2 c.	20 gm
Peanut Butter	2 tbsp.	9 gm
Cooked Cereals	3/4 c.	10-18 gm
Navy & Lima Beans	1 c.	6-8 gm
Bread	1 slice	2 gm
Nuts	1/2 c.	14-22 gm
Oatmeal	1 c.	5 gm
Collards	1 c.	5 gm
Lentils	1 c.	5 gm
Prunes	1 c.	3 gm
Frozen Peas	1 c.	5 gm
Chopped Nuts		
Almonds	1/3 c.	7 gm
Cashews	1 3/4 c.	7 gm
Peanuts	2 tbsp.	7 gm
Pecans	2/3 c.	7 gm
Walnuts	1/2 c.	7 gm
Worthington Foods		
Dinner Entree	2 oz.	7 gm
Protose	1 oz.	7 gm
Sandwich Spread	2 oz.	7 gm
Soy Beans/Sauce	2 oz.	7 gm

Protein Requirements Daily: Men — 52 grams; Women — 44 grams; Ages 1-12 — 23 grams. The larger the frame, the more protein required. Authorities differ as to daily requirement.

The Truth About Sugar

Recently a group of dieticians published a pamphlet on the harmful effects of excessive sugar consumption. They began with this fascinating sentence: "Judging by the size of America's sugar bowl, it really ought to be a sweet world." Imagine the United States map as a great bowl of sugar, filled up with Hershey Bars and peanut brittle and hard candy and gum drops and jelly beans and ice cream and sugar of all sorts. Someone has said, "Every day in America is sweeter than the day before," and it is! We're eating more and more sugar all the time. According to a survey by the U.S. Department of Agriculture, Americans eat approximately 3,500,000 pounds of candy each year. That's about 16 lbs. for every man, woman, and child in the country. This is only the beginning of the story. America's sweet tooth gets longer each year. Our craving for sweets seems to be more intense with each passing decade. Each American consumes approximately 120 lbs. of sugar per year. In the last 170 years, that increase in sugar has been remarkable.

In 1822 the average American ate two teaspoons of sugar a day; in 1890 — 10 teaspoons per day; in 1905 — 20 teaspoons per day. By 1974 the average American ate 33 teaspoons per day. In the 1990s the average American will eat approximately 40 teaspoons per day.

What is this excessive amount of sugar doing to our health, and where does this sugar come from? Let's take a look at the sugar consumption in our diet.

Where Is All This Sugar Coming From?

You're probably thinking, "Says who? I'm not getting that amount of sugar in my diet. Certainly I don't eat 40 teaspoons of sugar a day... or 120 pounds a year!" Are you aware of the fact that one piece of chewing gum has a half teaspoon of sugar, a glazed donut — six teaspoons, three scoops of ice cream — 12 teaspoons, a banana split — 24 teaspoons of sugar? Every piece of candy is 75% to 80% sugar. Popular candy bars weighing just five ounces usually contain 15 to 20 teaspoons of sugar. So the next time you pick up that Hershey bar, begin to scoop out your sugar — one, two, three, four, five, and count up to 20 teaspoons.

Most people aren't aware of the large amounts of sugar they are consuming because it is hidden in the foods they eat. The common conception is: "Someone else must be getting my share. Certainly I'm not eating that much sugar." A more careful analysis indicates that most of us are. Even some foods promoted as "health foods" have large amounts of sugar. Nature Valley "Fruit and Nut Granola" is 29% sugar, while Country Morning "Breakfast Cereal" is 31% sugar. Even General Mills "Raisin Bran" runs at 30.4% sugar. What could be more healthy than something called "Apple Jacks"? There is no problem with the apples! The problem is the enormous amount of added sugar — 54%. Ouch! That means that over half the dry contents in that bowl are sugar!

What is all this sugar doing to our bodies? How does it affect us? Is excessive sugar consumption all that bad?

Health Hazards of a High-Sugar Diet

What are some of the health hazards of a high-sugar diet? Is sugar something that is simply a quick energy food with no harmful effects on the body? The Seventh-day Adventist Dietetic Association, discussing sugar, said: "Highly refined sugar contains no nutrients except sucrose which is digested rapidly and the products are readily absorbed into the system. The fast rate of absorption is the reason why sugar has a reputation of being a quick energy food." Many people associate sugar with health, because it is a quick source of energy.

There are several problems, however, with this quick absorption of sucrose. Since carbohydrates require a number of B-vitamins for the body to process them, and sugar contains no B-vitamins, the body must draw on its reserves, leaving the possibility of a vitamin B deficiency. High sugar intake has also been associated with obesity, tooth decay, heart disease, diabetes, infection, and irritability. Let's examine these five health-destroying effects of excessive sugar more closely.

Obesity — The average American gets 20% of his/her calories from the 120 lbs. of sugar he/she eats each year. Many people find it easier to overeat refined, concentrated foods. It's hard to eat four apples, but not difficult to eat a bag of potato chips or maybe two. It's difficult to eat four bananas, not hard to eat four candy bars. The more you concentrate food, the more you sweeten food, the easier it becomes to absorb excessive amounts of calories. Sugar calories not used by the body are stored as fat. Since obesity contributes to heart disease, sugar can be a major culprit.

If you want to cut down on your weight, cut down on excessive sugars, particularly sugars that are eaten between meals. We're not suggesting that you cut out all desserts. There are some wonderful healthy dessert recipes in this book! But if you do eat dessert, if you eat pie or cake, be sure to eat a moderate amount once, or at most, twice a week. Eat it only after a meal, and never in between meals.

Tooth decay in children is promoted by excessive sugar eating. This sugar is easily fermented by bacteria in the mouth. Experimental animals on a high-sugar diet are observed to have blocked fluid movement in the canals of the teeth, causing rapid deterioration.

Due to the effect of World War II, Norway had a significant reduction in its supply of sugar. This decrease in sugar supply caused a reduction in sugar consumption which continued from 1939 to 1945. During the war years, a 70% reduction in tooth decay was noted.

You know, in Alaska an amazing 600% increase in tooth decay was reported by Dr. T.J. Pyle, Dental Supervisor at a school there, one year after the opening of the student snack bar canteen in which 28,000 candy bars were sold. If you want to increase your children's tooth decay — and your dental bills — increase the amount of sugar they eat.

Heart disease is a third health problem that is increased by high levels of sugar in the diet. Although there are many risk factors contributing to coronary artery disease, excessive sugar consumption has been implicated as one possible risk factor. There are many others — lack of exercise, smoking, high stress levels, high blood pressure, obesity, and so forth. But sugar consumption appears to be a contributing factor to coronary heart disease, particularly when combined with a high-fat diet.

Dr. Yudkin's studies at the University of London found that men who suffered heart attacks ate twice as much sugar in their diet as other men. Investigators have discovered that fat and sugar together tend to elevate fatty substances much higher than either one alone. For example, when you go out and eat a hamburger, french fries — both high in saturated fats — and combine that with ice cream, which is also high in fat and high in sugar, that becomes extremely detrimental to the heart and bloodstream.

Body Chemistry and a High-Sugar Diet

Some people suffer from hypoglycemia or low blood sugar. Many physicians are currently leaning toward the idea that America's excessive eating of sugar, especially between meals, tends to cause the blood sugar levels to rapidly rise, then fall quickly below the normal levels. The high of quick energy is followed by a corresponding low of tiredness and lethargy. This is true of all stimulants, and can contribute to low blood sugar or hypoglycemia.

Probably one of the more significant studies that has been done in the area of sugar and sugar consumption is in regard to infection or susceptibility to disease. Have you ever noticed that children often have more colds around the holidays? Have you noticed as well that when you give kids a diet high in sugar they may become more irritable? Why is it that there is a greater susceptibility to disease and irritability in children on a high-sugar diet? When there is danger of infection, the white blood cells increase in number in the blood stream. These soldiers of the body destroy bacteria, the infection causing agent. But when the blood sugar level goes up, they become sluggish and cannot destroy as many bacteria.

Loma Linda University has done some significant research on sugar and its relationship to disease. The researchers have discovered that there is a significant temporary decrease in the ability of certain white blood cells, the phagocytes, to destroy bacteria after a person eats a large amount of sugar at one time.

Normal levels of white blood cell activity do not return until five to six hours later. For example, if an individual has eaten no sugar at all, the number of bacteria destroyed by each white blood cell in 30 minutes is 14. If they have eaten, for example, six teaspoons of sugar, the number of bacteria destroyed is 10. If they've eaten 12 teaspoons, the number of bacteria destroyed in 30 minutes is 5.5. If they've eaten 18 teaspoons of sugar, the number of bacteria destroyed in 30 minutes is one! It's astounding to recognize that there is a major reduction in the ability of the body to fight off disease. [Notice the chart on the following page.]

This is why children who eat a lot of sweets are particularly vulnerable to colds and infections. Their white blood cell system, their phagocytes (cells that destroy invading sickness), are reduced. So they miss school and do more poorly in their grades. Consequently, they spend more time at the doctor and have higher dentist bills. They also become more irritable.

Sugars also appear to be habit forming — the more a person eats, the more they want. This presents a problem since sugar is replacing the more nutritious, balanced foods.

You see, excessive sugar and the lack of vitamin B complex and certain minerals result in the incomplete metabolism of sugar to carbon dioxide and cause pyruvic acid buildup. When pyruvic acid builds up there is a neutralization of vitamin B, resulting in irritability. For

Effect of Sugar Intake on the Ability of White Blood Cells (WBC) to Destroy Bacteria		
Teaspoons of sugar eaten at one time by an average adult	Number of bacteria destroyed by each WBC in 30 min.	Percentage decrease in ability to destroy bacteria
0	14	0
6	10	25
12	5.5	60
18	1	85
24	1	92

example, little Johnny sits down to that great birthday meal and quickly rushes through the pizza to get to the big-time cake, eating two pieces with three scoops of ice cream. This is why you can hardly control Johnny when the party is over. His nerves are frayed. He's anxious, tense, and uptight. Not only is Johnny climbing the walls, but mom is climbing the walls right along with him! If you'd like your children to remain more calm, less irritable, less hypertensive, less high-strung, reduce the amount of sugar in their diet.

What are some ways to do this?

How to Change a High-Sugar Diet

Let me give you some examples of a way you may be able to replace artificial sweets with natural ones. Look at the following chart: Rather than chocolate cake, why don't you try a carob cake. Carob is a natural food product and doesn't have the harmful effects that chocolate has. Chocolate has theobromine in it, which serves as a stimulant similar to caffeine. Carob cake would be much more healthful.

Rather than chocolate chip cookies, try some carob chip cookies or applesauce cookies. Instead of glazed donuts, how about whole wheat blueberry or raisin bagels? Rather than soda pop, try some lovely fruit juices. Fruit juices are particularly nice in the evening with a lighter fruit meal.

Rather than hard candy, which is 75% sugar, sample some dried fruits. Rather than sweet pies, which contain over 50% sugar, serve up fruit pies — apple, blueberry, strawberry pie. What about ice cream, which not only often contains excessive amounts of sugar, but also excessive amounts of fats and artificial preservatives and chemicals? Instead, make your own homemade soy ice cream or fruit sherbets. Make it a family affair, with the whole family participating on a Saturday night, cranking up healthful, delicious, and really nice-tasting ice cream.

What's the bottom line? Nutritional research continues to produce evidence that the imbalance in the American diet is causing an alarming increase in degenerative diseases. Our sugar and fat consumption is far too high. It's just killing us! Dr. Rodger J. Williams, a biochemist, has spent thirty years in research on the nutrition of a single cell. (He is the discoverer of pantothenic acid, one of the B-vitamins, and former president of the American Chemical Society.) He's looked at a single cell, and wondered, "How does it grow? How does protein in the cell affect it? How do the nutrients eaten by the body affect the life and growth of a cell?"

Dr. Williams observes: "Malnutrition — unbalanced or inadequate nutrition — at the cellular level should be thought of as a major cause of human disease. This seems crystal clear to me." This distinguished scientist sàys that if there is inadequate nutrition, there will be destruction on the cellular level. This destruction could, of course, predispose us to heart disease or cancer. Dr. Williams makes a significant point here.

Our body was designed to assimilate the nutrients from a wide variety of wholesome foods. It wasn't designed for "junk foods" high in fat and sugar and refined artificially. One of the reasons scores of children, youth, and adults are so often hungry and constantly eating without being satisfied is because of what some nutritionists call "hidden hunger" — the body's craving for wholesome foods. The more "junk foods" a person eats, the more their body cries out for nutritious foods. There is something missing inside. There's a craving for wheat bread, fruits, nuts, grains, and vegetables Some of our suggested lentil and bean dishes would satisfy that craving! There is a desire inside the body for fresh fruits and vegetables, and a desire for healthy desserts.

Have you ever noticed that if you're eating, and you're a little full, but you then eat a sugar dessert, you still seem to have a hidden hunger that's not satisfied? This is because artificial sweeteners such as sugar stimulate the body to require more food. This contributes to obesity because the "hidden hunger" of the body hasn't been satisfied. As you feed your family wholesome, nutritious meals, they will be truly satisfied. The constant nibbling to fill up that hole will be replaced with a sense of satisfied wholeness. Your family will anticipate meals, enjoy them, and reap the benefits of good health.

Chapter
6

The Joy of Natural Cooking

The ancient Scriptures declare: "Beloved, above all things, I pray that you would prosper and be in health as your soul prospers." 3 John 2. In our last chapter, we talked about "hidden hunger," that desire of the body to be nourished by wholesome foods. But there is another form of "hidden hunger." One noted psychiatrist affirmed, "Man acts better, lives better, does better and responds better if he believes in God." He pointed out that there is an emptiness in every heart. Every human being has it — a hunger for God. There is a God-shaped vacuum within each of our hearts that only our Creator can satisfy. Humans are physical, mental, and spiritual beings. Health consists of total well-being. It is physical well-being, mental alertness, and spiritual harmony or peace.

Our wish for you is a life of abundant physical health, filled with zest, vitality, and energy. We wish you a life of mental joy, inner peace, and happy relationships with those around you. The greatest desire for you is a spiritual openness with the God who created you and longs to be your Best Friend. Maybe there are things in your life that aren't satisfying to you. Maybe there's an empty longing inside. I suggest that you not only prepare healthful recipes, but on your knees, you ask this God to be your Friend.

Enjoy the following recipes and guidelines, and reap the benefits of good health!

Ten Steps to Successful Breadmaking

I. Recipe
  A. Choose a simple, basic recipe.
  B. If you are a beginner in breadmaking, it would be helpful to use soy, gluten, or unbleached white flour with the whole wheat flour.

II. Yeast
  A. Kinds of yeast:
    1. dry yeast — added directly to dry flour.
    2. dry active yeast — softened in warm water (110°).
    3. compressed or fresh yeast — softened in lukewarm water (85°).
  B. Factors that retard yeast:
    1. Salt and fat retard the growth of the yeast and should not be added to a yeast mixture until it has grown very active by feeding on sugar and starch.
    2. Too much sugar added directly to the yeast may somewhat retard the action.
    3. Dry active yeast that is too old will retard growth.

III. Mixing
  A. Mix ingredients — water, sweetening, salt, and oil. Add different kinds of flours to change the kind of bread.
  B. Develop the gluten of the wheat flour in the batter by beating thoroughly, then add other kinds of flour.
  C. Bread of fine texture and good flavor is partly the result of thorough kneading after all the ingredients have been combined.
  D. Other ingredients in addition to the flour, like raisins, apricots, caraway seeds, etc., should be added to the basic ingredients while they are still a liquid. Then enough flour is added to obtain a stiff dough.

IV. Kneading
  A. All the flour necessary to keep dough from sticking to your hands should be added at the time of kneading. (A poor job of kneading dough before the first rising cannot be remedied.)

B. A good way to knead is to lift the dough with fingers, fold it over and push down with the heel of the hand. Do this over and over until you have a smooth ball.

V. Rising

A. Place dough in oiled bowl. Cover to prevent forming crust.

B. Let rise in warm place (not hot) until double in size (about 1½ hours).

VI. Making Loaves

A. Punch down, divide and form into balls.

B. Use approximately 1 to 1¼ pounds of dough to each loaf.

C. The loaf will take the shape of the pan so don't fill pans too full or bread will spill over the sides causing cracked, over-browned crusts.

D. Form into loaves and place in bread pan.

VII. Rising in Bread Pans

A. Let rise 45 minutes to 1 hour before baking.

B. When bread is doubled in bulk and ready to bake, dough will retain a dent when pressed lightly.

C. Over-raised bread can fall when it hits the extreme heat, so it is better to bake a little "under" raised than "over" raised.

VIII. Baking

A. Bake in moderate oven 350° F.

B. Bake until thoroughly done — approximately 40 to 45 minutes.

C. Loaves should be golden brown on all sides.

D. Bread should slip out of the pan easily if baked properly.

IX. Cooling

A. Leave uncovered on racks.

B. Cool thoroughly before putting into bags.

X. Storing

A. Homemade bread will keep approximately one week stored in bread box.

B. Bread freezes well. Make several different kinds and freeze.

[When using the following recipes, persons on a low-fat diet may choose to reduce or eliminate fats.]

BREAD RECIPES

100% WHOLE WHEAT BREAD

2 packages active dry yeast
$1/4$ cup warm water
$2^1/2$ cups hot water
$1/4$ to $1/2$ cup honey
1 T. salt
$1/4$ cup oil
1 cup wheat germ
7 cups whole wheat flour

SOFTEN active dry yeast in $1/4$ cup warm water.
COMBINE hot water, honey, salt, and oil in another
    bowl.
STIR in wheat germ.
ADD 4 cups whole wheat flour to make a moderately
    stiff dough.
ADD softened yeast mixture to dough.
ADD remaining flour.
TURN OUT on a lightly floured surface.
KNEAD until smooth and satiny.
SHAPE dough into a ball.
PLACE in lightly greased bowl.
COVER and let rise in a warm place until double
    (about $1^1/2$ hours).

PUNCH down.

CUT into 2 portions (about 1¼ to 1½ lbs. each).

SHAPE each into smooth ball.

SHAPE into loaves.

LET RISE until double (about 1 hour).

BAKE 30-35 minutes at 350° F.

DANISH SWEET ROLLS

2 packages active dry yeast

¼ cup warm water

2½ cups water

½ cup brown sugar

1 T. salt

¼ cup oil

1 cup oatmeal

½ cup wheat germ

3 cups whole wheat flour

4 cups unbleached white flour

SOFTEN active yeast in ¼ cup warm water.

MIX ingredients together. (Follow same instructions as Whole Wheat Bread for making bread dough.)

LET rise.

PUNCH down after first rising of about 1½ hours.

ROLL OUT in 3 sections.

BRUSH dough with 2 T. melted butter.

SPRINKLE on 2 T. brown sugar.

COMBINE $^1/_3$ cup raisins and nuts.
SPREAD on dough.
ROLL as for jelly roll.
SHAPE in ring.
PLACE on baking dish.
CUT almost to center.
COVER and let rise about 50 minutes.
BAKE at 350^0 F. for about 25-30 minutes.

BREAKFAST RECIPES

GRANOLA

7 cups oatmeal
1 cup wheat germ
1 cup coconut (finely ground)
1 $^1/_2$ t. salt
1 cup slivered almonds or chopped
   pecans, etc.
$^1/_4$ to $^1/_2$ cup oil
$^1/_2$ cup warm water
$^1/_4$ to $^1/_2$ cup honey
1 t. vanilla

MIX above dry ingredients together in large pan.
ADD liquid to dry ingredients.
MIX thoroughly.
PUT in large shallow pans.
BAKE at 225^0 F. until golden brown and crisp
   (about 2 to 2$^1/_2$ hours) or bake slowly at 170^0 F.
   for 6-7 hours.

SERVE with fruit, if desired. Fresh peaches, strawberries, or fruit puree are especially delicious.

BAKED OATMEAL

4 cups water
1 t. salt
3 cups oats
$\frac{1}{2}$ cup coconut
$\frac{1}{4}$ cup chopped dates
2 T. oil (optional)

BOIL water and salt.
MIX remaining ingredients.
ADD water all at once.
BAKE in shallow dish at 375° F. for 30-40 minutes.

APRICOT JAM

2 cups dried apricots
Unsweetened pineapple juice

SOAK dried apricots in unsweetened pineapple juice until soft.
ADD enough juice to cover apricots.
BLEND into a jam.

APPLE CRISP

6 to 8 large apples, peeled and sliced
2 cups unsweetened pineapple juice
2-3 T. cornstarch

2 cups rolled oats
1 cup whole wheat flour
$^1/_4$ cup wheat germ
$^1/_4$ cup nuts
$^1/_4$ cup brown sugar
$^1/_4$ t. salt
1 t. vanilla
$^1/_2$ cup oil
$^1/_4$ cup water

PLACE peeled and sliced apples in bottom of Pyrex
   baking dish.
THICKEN unsweetened pineapple juice with cornstarch.
POUR this mixture over apples.
MIX remaining ingredients thoroughly in a bowl.
SPREAD over sliced apples in shallow pan.
BAKE until golden brown in moderate oven
   (350^0 F.) approximately 30 minutes.

Variations: Use this topping on other fresh fruit and berries, or on
thickened peaches or other canned fruit.

MAIN MEAL RECIPES

CASHEW NUT LOAF

1 cup onion, chopped
1½ cups celery, chopped
2 cans mushroom soup
2 cans water
2 envelopes George Washington
   Broth*
1½ cups cashews
2 cans (5 oz.) Chinese noodles

MIX all ingredients together.
PLACE in casserole dish.
BAKE at 350⁰ F. for about 1 hour.

*Buy in health food store or substitute a seasoning broth.

VEGETABLE POT PIE

2 cups potatoes, diced small
1½ cups carrots, diced small
½ small onion, chopped
1 package frozen peas
1 cup gluten or textured vegetable
   protein

Cream Sauce:
2 T. flour   2 cups soy milk
2 T. oil   2 t. vegetable stock

STEAM potatoes, carrots, onion, until tender.
ADD vegetable protein and peas.
MIX lightly.
PLACE this mixture in casserole dish.

COMBINE Cream Sauce ingredients.
COOK together on low to medium heat, stirring
    constantly until thickened.
POUR over vegetables in casserole dish.
COVER with pie crust.
BAKE in hot oven, 425-450° F. for 20 minutes or until
    nicely browned.

WHEAT GERM PATTIES

$1^1/_2$ cups wheat germ
1 cup uncooked oatmeal
$^1/_2$ cup chopped nuts
4 t. soy sauce
$^1/_2$ t. salt
$^1/_4$ t. sage
1 clove garlic or 1 t. garlic powder
1 medium onion, minced
1 cup soy milk

MIX well.
FORM into patties.
BROWN both sides in oil.
PLACE in baking dish.
COVER with mushroom soup or tomato sauce.
BAKE at 350° F. for 10 to 15 minutes.

CHOW MEIN

2 T. oil
2 cups peeled onion, sliced
1 cup sliced gluten

2 cups celery, sliced
1 green pepper, sliced
1 can water chestnuts, drained, sliced
    or ½ cup raw cashew nuts
1 can bean sprouts, drained
1 or 2 T. soy sauce or Bragg Liquid
    Aminos*
1 cup water
2 T. cornstarch

SAUTE onions, and gluten in oil.
ADD and COOK remaining ingredients quickly, stirring
    constantly.
THICKEN with cornstarch mixed with a little water.
SERVE over rice.

*Buy in health food store. This is an unfermented soy
sauce with no added salt.

GLUTEN AND GLUTEN BROTH

Gluten:
8 cups whole wheat flour
4 cups water

Broth:
2 qts. water
1 onion, diced
1 T. Vegex
$\frac{1}{2}$ t. garlic powder
$\frac{1}{3}$ c. soy sauce
2 T. oil (optional)

MIX flour and water.
KNEAD thoroughly.
COVER dough entirely with water.
LET SOAK for at least 1 hour.
WASH or rinse thoroughly, keeping the dough together.
CONTINUE working the dough in water until you have a
    tough elastic lump which is mainly gluten, the
    protein of the wheat.
SLICE gluten into steak-like pieces and add to boiling
    broth.
SIMMER until most of liquid is gone.

Remaining broth may be thickened into a gravy and
served over gluten steaks. Gluten may be breaded and
baked, or browned in skillet.

LENTIL STEW

$^1/_2$ cup celery, chopped
1 onion, chopped
1 cup carrots, sliced
2 cups potatoes, diced
1 cup dry lentils
1 t. salt
2 T. parsley
1 qt. water
1 can tomatoes (1 lb., 12 oz.),
   chopped
$^1/_4$ t. thyme

PLACE all ingredients (except tomatoes) in saucepan.
COOK on low heat for about 1 hour.
ADD tomatoes to cook last 15 minutes.

OATBURGERS

$4^1/_2$ cups water
$^1/_2$ cup soy sauce
$4^1/_2$ cups oats
1 onion, chopped
1 t. garlic powder
$^1/_4$ cup Brewers yeast
2 T. oil

BRING water, soy sauce, and seasoning to a boil.
TURN DOWN heat.

ADD onion and oats.

FORM into patties.

BAKE until nicely browned at 350⁰ F. for about
45 minutes.

TURN after 20 minutes.

DESSERT RECIPES

DATE LAYER BARS

$1/2$ cups margarine
$1/2$ cup brown sugar
$1^1/2$ cups unbleached white flour
1 t. salt
$1^1/2$ cups quick-cooking rolled oats
1 T. wheat germ
$1/2$ cup nuts
1 T. water
1 recipe date filling (see below)

Filling:
2 cups pitted dates
2 cups water

CREAM together margarine and sugar.

STIR dry ingredients into creamed mixture.

ADD water and MIX until crumbly.

FIRMLY PAT one-half of the mixture into greased baking
dish.

SPREAD with date filling.

TOP with remaining crumbs.
PAT smooth.
BAKE at 350^0 F. for about 30 minutes.

Date Filling:
COMBINE ingredients in saucepan.
COVER.
COOK, stirring often until consistency of jam.
ADD more water as needed.

APPLESAUCE COOKIES

$1/2$ cup honey or brown sugar
$1/2$ cup oil
1 cup applesauce
$1/2$ cup chopped nuts
$1/2$ t. salt
1 t. vanilla
4 cups quick oats

BEAT oil and sugar together until well blended.
ADD remaining ingredients.
MIX well.
DROP from teaspoon onto oiled cookie sheet.
BAKE at 325^0 F. for 20 to 25 minutes, or until nicely
      browned.
LET COOL before removing from cookie sheet.

CARROT PIE

1 cup dates
2$\frac{1}{2}$ T. cornstarch
$\frac{3}{4}$ t. salt
3 T. soy flour
1 t. vanilla
3 T. oil
1$\frac{3}{4}$ cups cooked carrots*
1$\frac{1}{2}$ cups soy milk

WHIZ all ingredients in blender.
POUR into pie plate that has been lined with crust.
BAKE at 350⁰ F. until set, about 35 minutes.
TOP with Soy Cream or whipped cream topping.

*Pumpkin or squash may be used in place or carrots.

DRIED FRUIT CANDY

2 cups dried apricots, ground
1 cup dates, ground
1 cup raisins, ground
$\frac{1}{2}$ cup nuts, crushed

MIX the above ingredients together.
FORM into small balls.
ROLL in $\frac{1}{2}$ cup crushed nuts

FRUIT DRINK RECIPES

FRUIT PUNCH

> 5 cups unsweetened pineapple
> juice, chilled
> 1 qt. apple juice, chilled
> 1 package (10 oz.) frozen
> strawberries, partially thawed
> 1 qt. sparkling mineral water
> Fresh strawberry slices
> Fresh lime slices

COMBINE pineapple and apple juices in punch bowl.
BLEND strawberries, undrained, in blender.
MIX into pineapple/apple juice.
POUR in mineral water just before serving.
GARNISH with strawberry and lime slices.

ORANGE BANANA DRINK

> 3 cups unsweetened pineapple juice
> 3 large bananas
> 2 (12 oz.) cans frozen orange juice
> 1 (12 oz.) can frozen lemonade

BLEND bananas with pineapple juice.
MIX with orange juice and lemonade, adding the amount
of water called for in frozen juices.

2000 and Beyond

Surviving Emotional Stress in the 90s

Imagine it's a beautiful starry night under the trees of the Sequoia National Park. You've just settled down for the night when you hear a rumbling outside your tent. Pretty soon your tent begins to shake. The tent pole falls, and rummaging around in the darkness, you sense that you're being attacked by a bear.

What happens in the body when a stressful situation like this occurs? The brain quickly recognizes an emergency and gives orders to the body to react in a manner appropriate to the seriousness of the situation. The "fight or flight" mechanism goes into motion. The brain arouses the sympathetic nervous system which deals with stress, and this system triggers the release of two hormones by the adrenal glands that let the body cells know the intensity of the stress. The pupils widen to enable you to see more. The blood vessels contract to allow for maximum efficiency. The heart beats faster, putting out more blood with each beat, which helps the muscles to work more strenuously. The diameter of the coronary arteries increases, allowing more room for the passage of the greater quantity of blood required by your heart.

The lungs react, too. The tiny air pipes of the lungs open wider. The rate and depth of breathing increase to allow more oxygen to be passed into the blood stream. The muscles receive more fuel and oxygen as the blood vessels within the muscles open wider.

Your state of mind has completely changed the physiological processes within your body. If a bear is chasing you, this is appropriate, especially if you are running for your life! But what if you feel like bears are chasing you all the time? What then happens to your body? What if you have nowhere to run and you feel the same level of stress? Let's see what effect positive and negative emotions have, and particularly the effect of stress as it relates to human physiology.

In the following pages you will learn what stress is and what it can do, but more importantly, you will learn how to manage it through the power of God's love. We trust that you will discover the joy of God's guidance and provision for your every need.

A government report reveals a new class of drug addicts in the United States — some 20 million women who suffer from dependency on pills and alcohol. In fact, Americans as a whole purchased more than 475 million dollars' worth of depressants or sedatives last year.

Why do thousands of Americans need daily doses of chemicals as a crutch? Why all the pill-popping and alcohol abuse at this particular point in time?

After discussing rising inflation, the growing lack of confidence in large government, and the average person's feeling of helplessness in controlling his own life, the editor of *Ambassador*, a Trans-World Airlines magazine, describes the problem this way: "It is in this bleak soil that the seeds of frustration and uncertainty have been planted, that the seeds of tension and discontent are growing. The hills are alive with the sound, not of music, but of split-level tempers and gripes from the ghettos. This widespread feeling that the quality of life isn't what it used to be a few years ago — and will never be again — has caused people to feel put upon, insecure, stressful, and emotionally unsure of themselves."

Obviously, the key to this matter of stress is in the way we think and approach the problems and challenges of life. Sedatives or depressants are designed to affect one's forebrain, one's thinking. A staff member at the Mayo Clinic is reported to have said, "We can deal with 25% of the people who come to us by the physical instrument of science; 75% we don't know what to do with, for they are passing on the sickness of their minds and their souls to their bodies."

A contributing factor of coronary heart disease is emotional stress. It is also a leading cause of stomach ulcers, tension headaches, rheumatoid arthritis, and various skin disorders.

Thinking influences bodily health. The mind and body function as a unit. Whatever affects thinking processes ultimately affects the body. Whatever affects the body (lack of sleep, overeating) eventually affects thinking. Hidden feelings may produce physical symptoms. The anxiety of the first day in a new school may cause a student to get sick to the point of vomiting. Business executives have been known to have a headache or possibly an attack of diarrhea before a speech. Performers or athletes may be so stressed that they lose their concentration and may not be able to do what they do normally without any problem in practice.

William C. Menninger, a noted authority in the field of mental health, stated it succinctly: "The organs of the body are just as much a part of the personality as is the mind. These organs are often used like mirrors, to reflect our feelings, like fear or anger." *Unbottled Poison*, p. 5.

The heart, the stomach, the liver and kidneys, are all "reflectors." They mirror our inner thoughts and feelings. The heart of the issue, then, is this: Our relationship to life's experiences must change if we are going to survive in the 90s.

Positive reactions to life's experiences produce positive chemical byproducts, while negative reactions to life's experiences produce negative byproducts.

In the best-seller book, *The Ministry of Healing*, p. 241, by Ellen G. White, she states: "Grief, anxiety, discontent, remorse, guilt, distrust, all tend to break down the life forces and to invite decay and death." No wonder Solomon said, "As... [a man] thinketh in his heart, so is he." Proverbs 23:7.

The circumstances of life or "stressors" do not in themselves produce stress. It's our reaction or relationship and attitude to them that produces tension. Thus, if we are going to have an effective strategy for stress control, it is imperative to develop positive emotions such as "gratitude, rejoicing, benevolence, trust [faith]... — these are health's greatest safeguard." *Ibid.*, p. 281.

An Effective Strategy For Stress Control

Being thankful is the first step. We will be happier and healthier and help make the world a better place to live in if we cultivate the habit of just being grateful and saying thank you. "Nothing tends more to promote health of body and of soul than does a spirit of gratitude and praise." *Ibid.*, p. 251.

There is a little song we sing from time to time in our home before meals. It goes like this:

"There is so much for which to be thankful,
There are gifts so abundant each day,
So we thank Thee, dear Lord, for Thy mercies,
Which attend us along life's way."

Develop an attitude of thankfulness, and it will go a long way toward reducing stress and keeping you well. We can learn to develop this thankful attitude when misfortune comes as well as when things run smoothly.

One day many years ago an English preacher traveling to a neighboring town on horseback was robbed. That evening, he made this entry in his journal:

"I was robbed today, yet I am thankful,
I am thankful first that, although they took all
I had, they really didn't take much.
I am thankful that, although they took my purse
they did not take my life.
Lastly, I am thankful that it was I who was robbed
and not I who robbed!"

Learn to give thanks continually. The sacred Scriptures give us this divine prescription: "In every thing give thanks: for this is the will of God in Christ Jesus concerning you." 1 Thessalonians 5:18.

The second step in our strategy for stress control is the ability to rejoice. It is a first cousin to thanksgiving. I'm not referring to a superficial giddiness, but to a deep, abiding happiness that is manifest continually in an attitude of rejoicing. Some time ago in *Reader's Digest* there appeared an article by Blake Clark on longevity. Mr. Clark interviewed a number of America's centenarians. In all of his interviews he found a common denominator: "Perhaps the key characteristic shared by most centenarians is a cheerful disposition, a feeling that things will work out for the best. ... Can serenity strengthen a cell, or tranquility erase a wrinkle? Who knows? But our centenarians, through their lives, tell us that songs and laughter somehow lubricate the biological clock and keep it running longer. Happiness, it appears, is the best preventive medicine." February, 1976, p. 132. Learn to smile, for as the wise man so aptly put it, "A merry heart doeth good like a medicine." Proverbs 17:22.

The third on the great quartet of positive emotions is benevolence. We improve our own health and the health of others when we practice simple kindness. If each of us were a little more thoughtful, a bit kinder, and more courteous each day to those at home, to those with whom we labor, and to those we meet, how much easier it would be to live in this stressful age.

Unselfishness is health-giving, while selfishness destroys health. Benevolence stimulates the life forces. Doing good for another benefits the doer more than the receiver. Ellen G. White wrote: "Good deeds are twice a blessing, benefiting both the giver and the receiver of the kindness. The consciousness of right-doing is one of the best medicines for diseased bodies and minds. When the mind is free and happy from a sense of duty well done and the satisfaction of giving happiness to others, the cheering, uplifting influence brings new life to the whole being." *The Ministry of Healing*, p. 257.

A few years ago, several medical researchers were studying the effect of the shocks of life on the central nervous system. They took one lamb and placed it in its pen alone. They hooked up electric shock devices around the pen. As the lamb wandered to one side of the pen, the researchers threw a switch and the lamb was shocked. Immediately it twitched and scampered to another part of the pen. Soon the researcher shocked the lamb again. Again he ran.

As the research continued, the scientists discovered that the lamb would never return to a place where previously he had been shocked. After a series of shocks, the little lamb stood in the center of his pen quivering. He had no place to run, nowhere to go. The shocks were everywhere. Completely overcome emotionally, filled with anxiety and stress, his nerves gave way.

The researchers then took this lamb's twin and placed it in a pen. This time, they put the lamb's mother in with him. Presently, they shocked him. Again the lamb ran, but this time he ran to his mother and snuggled up to her closely. Evidently she reassured him, because he left her side to begin eating again. The researchers threw the switch again, and once again the lamb ran to his mother. Reassuringly, she consoled him again. The researchers then noted a remarkable difference in the two lambs. The second lamb had no fear of returning to the spot where he received the shock. To the utter amazement of the researchers, future shocks no longer disturbed him. He showed none of the symptoms of nervousness, stress, or anxiety that his twin showed under the same circumstances. What made this remarkable difference? He had the assurance of someone to flee to in stress. He had confidence and power in someone outside of himself to cope with the stress.

Everyone needs to have such confidence. Even Julia Huxley, the infidel philosopher, admits, "Man does better if he believes as if God is there." There is a deep need within the human heart for someone in whom to place confidence, someone to whom one can go in trouble, someone who will offer reassurance in the stresses and strains of life.

The One who made us loves us and desires to soothe our frayed nerves, ease our restless longings, and calm our anxieties. Because He made us, we matter to Him. Long ago Jesus gave this beautiful invitation, "Come unto me, all ye that labor and are heavy laden, and I will give you rest. Take my yoke upon you, and learn of me. . . .: and ye shall find rest unto your souls." Matthew 11:28, 29. True rest is found in a loving trust relationship with our Creator. Down through the centuries of time Christ's gentle invitation remains the same, "Come unto me, . . . I will give you rest."

Learn by personal experience the rewards and satisfactions of claiming the promises of God. The following are examples of promises to be claimed in times of:

a. anxiety — Matthew 6:31-34
b. fear — Psalm 23; Psalm 91; Psalm 43:1, 2
c. indecision — James 1:5-7; Jeremiah 33:3
d. restlessness — John 14:27; Psalm 119:165;
   Philippians 4:6, 7
e. sleeplessness — Psalm 4:8
f. guilt — 1 John 1:9
g. loneliness — Matthew 28:20; Isaiah 49:15, 16
h. misfortune — Malachi 3:10, 11; Psalm 46:1
i. depression — Jeremiah 31:13; Psalm 126:5, 6
j. sickness — James 5:14, 15
k. discouragement — Psalm 27:14